The Flexible Diet Ultimate Guide!

Flexible Diet

Weight Loss Has Never Been Easier! - Get Lean Fast The Simple Way With This IIFYM Flexible Dieting Guide To Fat Loss Forever!

Chris Smith

Copyright © 2015 Chris Smith

STOP!!! Before you read any further....Would you like to know the Secrets of Body Transformation?

If your answer is yes, then you are not alone. Thousands of people are looking for the secret to rapidly burn body fat, keep the weight off, become healthier, and truly transform their body and life for good.

If you have been searching for these answers without much luck, you are in the right place!

Not only will you gain incredible insight in this book, but because I want to make sure to give you as much value as possible, right now for a limited time you can get full **100% FREE access to a VIP bonus EBook** entitled **THE 7 KEYS TO BODY TRANSFORMATION!**

Just Go Here For Free Instant Access:

www.liveFitVIP.com

Legal Notice

Disclaimer Notice

Table Of Contents

Introduction

I want to thank you and congratulate you for purchasing the book, *"Flexible Diet: The Flexible Diet Ultimate Guide! - Weight Loss Has Never Been Easier! - Get Lean Fast The Simple Way With This IIFYM Flexible Dieting Guide To Fat Loss Forever!*

This book contains proven steps and strategies on how to loss fat forever.

The primary concern of most dieters is that they are having a hard time controlling their selves from eating the food they want. Most of the diet programs restrict the dieter's food intake thus resulting from unhealthy way of losing fat. With IIFYM, you can eat the food that you want and at the same time gain the muscle that you want and lose those unwanted fats. This book will guide you how to do the Flexible Dieting without affecting your everyday activities. Definitely, this book will help you get in shape long term.

Thanks again for purchasing this book, I hope you enjoy it!

Chapter 1 - What Is Flexible Dieting?

The process of tracking the carbohydrate, fat and protein intake to change the body composition is Flexible Dieting. Also known as , "If It Fits Your Macros" or IIFYM, this is a simple way to losing weight that focuses on your daily intake of calories and the macronutrient content of your food choices. Although this idea has been around for many years, it has only recently that its popularity exploded.

IIFYM is a dieting method made to fit any kind of lifestyle. You can eat any kind of food that you want without going off target, while still completing your daily calorie and macronutrient goals. This type of dieting helps create a healthy connection with food and eliminates the worries attached to going on a traditional diet. You no longer have to feel guilty about eating the "wrong" kinds of foods because there is no such thing in IIFYM. Now that you don't feel guilty most of the time, you will be able to focus on the program and actually lose weight more efficiently.

The difference between traditional diets and flexible dieting is the former focuses on minimizing calorie intake not the kinds of food you get it from. Weight loss can actually happen in a short amount of time by excluding calories altogether. However, the urge to eat will come back and it will be stronger than before, you will not be able to stop yourself from eating and you will regain all the weight you lost, and maybe even gain a bit more. IIFYM or Flexible dieting is a long-term plan; it is easy enough that you can lose your excess weight and keep it off forever.

In order to lose weight you need to determine your daily calorie requirement. Then you analyze your macronutrient goals – in other words, you need to find out how much carbohydrates, fat and protein you need to consume every day. You will then eat only the foods that bring you to those numbers – hence the name, IIFYM- If it Fits Your Macros.

The Macronutrients

Macros or macronutrients, compose the biggest part of our daily diet, they are:

Carbohydrates

Carbs constitute the biggest part of your daily diet. In fixed diets, you are told to avoid carbohydrates as much as possible. However, you do not need to concern yourself about carb intake too much when you are on a flexible diet. Your goal is to add several parts of fibrous vegetables and fruit every day to counteract the excess carbs.

Protein

This macro is important for muscle growth and maintenance. Proteins are usually less important in conventional diets, but in flexible dieting, it is one of the focal points.

Fat

Fats play an essential role in keeping the hair and skin healthy, and it is essential for the production of hormones that affects your moods. You don't have to identify the types of fat, just make sure you meet your overall fat target.

Compare the Macronutrients

Here is an example of how you can compare macros: people consider salads as healthy while a donut is not, but if you break them down to their macronutrient content, they are actually the same. Our body doesn't have the capability of identifying which foods we eat are healthy and which has fewer nutrients. As long as your diet contains the right amount of fiber and macronutrients then you can eat anything you want.

Chapter 2 - How To Do Flexible Dieting

As mentioned in the first chapter, the flexible diet focuses on macronutrients. This chapter will discuss how to do the flexible diet the right way and achieve the healthy body that you want.

1. Calculate your Everyday Calorie Requirements

You will base your daily calorie requirement on your Basal Metabolic Rate, which in turn depends on your everyday physical activities; this will provide you with a rough estimate of your TDEE or Total Daily Energy Expenditure. In order to lose weight, you need fewer calories, and to add weight you need to increase them.

Your daily protein requirements depends on your goal; an average individual may target a 0.65g/lb body weight to retain the muscle mass, while weight lifters and athletes aims for 1g/lb. Fats form 25% of your calories, the remaining calories are carbohydrates. You should also aim to achieve the recommended mineral and vitamin requirements and at least 1.4g of fiber for every 1,000 calories.

2. Track Your Diet

Tracking calories and macronutrient intake is much easier than before. Nowadays there are apps that will scan the barcode of foods and tell you the amount of macronutrients they contain. You can also use a kitchen scale to measure the amount of food you eat so you know exactly how much food is going into your body. Tracking how much food and what kinds of food you eat are important in flexible dieting.

3. Weighing In

Just like traditional diets, you need to keep track of your weight on a regular basis. You are required to weigh yourself every day then get the weekly average, by doing this you can make sure that you are not losing or gaining weight too slowly or quickly, because this often leads to hazardous weight fluctuations. If you want to lose weight in a healthy manner then you need to aim for 1-2 pounds weight loss every week and vice versa if you want to gain weight.

4. Making Adjustments

If there are no changes in your weight then you may need to make small adjustments in a gradual manner. For instance, if after a week or so of dieting and your weight remains unchanged then you need to lower your calories intake to 50 each day. Your calories should come from carbs and fats, while keeping the same amount of protein. Continue lowering your carb consumption slightly until you start seeing the numbers on the scale wind down at an acceptable rate. It is also worth saying that as you gain or lose weight while on your diet your calorie consumption may change.

5. Transitioning Between Phases

Once you achieve your goal at every stage of your diet, you need to transition properly towards the next stage. Sudden change in your weight is not healthy for your body since it greatly affects your metabolism. Changing your calorie intake right away from low consumption to high could lead to weight gain again. Make sure to maintain your calorie intake at roughly the same amount as when you were seeing positive weight loss results.

If you want to add muscles and not just lose weight, increase your calories slowly week by week to have a healthy transition between phases. Check yourself in the mirror every once in a while to make sure that you are in fact gaining muscle mass, not fat. This could be a slow process, but it is important to make sure that you don't fall into a dangerous yo-yo weight loss cycle.

Chapter 3 - Understanding IIFYM (If It Fits Your Macros)

"IIFYM" or "If It Fits Your Macros" is a diet program to enhance your body composition by taking the right amount of calories and other macronutrients. The brain, heart and other vital organs are not addressed in the IIFYM and it also does not focus on healthy eating.

In a flexible diet, if you eat fewer amounts of calories than what your body requires, you will lose weight at a steady and expected rate. It makes fat loss much easier. All you need to do is to maintain your daily macros and the fats will start melting away gradually.

The Origins of IIFYM

A group of competitive bodybuilders who got tired of eating "bro" and "clean foods" to keep fit in between competitions accidentally discovered IIFYM. The traditional bodybuilder's diet is very plain, tasteless and has very few options when it comes to food. The conventional diet includes the following:

- Chicken and turkey breast
- Steamed vegetables
- Brown rice
- Oats or plain oatmeal
- Egg whites
- Protein Shakes

These "clean foods" are bland and boring. Many dieters got tired of eating "boring foods" which eventually led to them giving up on their weight loss aspirations. Surely, the conventional diet has been helping athletes lose weight for many years, but it also made their life miserable. Thanks to the athletes who inadvertently came up with the IIFYM method of dieting, bodybuilders and athletes can eat the foods they want and still lose weight. In IIFYM you are allowed to eat foods such as:

- Buffalo Wings

- Candy
- Cheesecake
- Cookies
- Donuts
- Fast food
- French fries
- Fried chicken
- Ice cream
- Pizza
- Pop Tarts

You can eat anything you want If It Fits Your Macros.

The IIFYM Connections

When people plan to lose weight, the first thing that enters their mind is that they need to clean up their diet. This may be true with some diet programs but not with IIFYM.

Eating clean, healthy food may help burn fats and lose weight, but there is no magical connection between losing weight and health food. One of the reasons why eating clean burns fat is because you are minimizing the amount of calories you eat, and getting rid of sweets, fried foods, and sauces, will certainly do just that. However, you need to reduce your calorie intake gradually. A sudden drop can significantly affect your metabolism, or at a minimum lessen metabolic capacity, which makes maintaining long-term weight loss much harder, and in some cases almost impossible.

The way you look depends on the amount of calories you take, thus if you eat clean, you lose weight. However, it is not the only answer to lose weight, it's just another technique that will help reduce fats much faster. The primary concern of eating clean and not monitoring the amount of calorie you take is that you end up starving yourself. This would cause the metabolism to bounce back. As a result, you not only regain the weight you lost, you also got a few more extra pounds when you start eating normal again.

People have this wrong notion that in order to lose weight, they need to starve themselves. You probably heard it from some fraud diet program, saying that you discredit calorie counting, and then offer you a diet plan or an item. After all, if they were able to tell you that monitoring calories equates to starvation, they might be able to convince you to purchase whatever products they are offering.

IIFYM does not encourage self-imposed starvation, nor does it tell you to eat as much "bad" foods as you want. It actually teaches you how to stay in between those two extremes so you can effectively lose weight.

Chapter 4 - How To Get Lean Fat Through IIFYM

If your main goal is to gain some serious muscle, you need to bulk up. Unless you are new at weightlifting or you have a very special genetic makeup, it is virtually impossible to lose weight and gain muscle at the same time. You need to watch your calories, this means eating more food than you actually need.

A bulk helps you get the muscle and fat. Gaining muscle without gaining fat is impossible if you are in a calorie surplus, which is around 5-10% of your daily requirement. However, to maintain the fat gain to a minimum, you should count your macros and you do your workouts effectively. Monitor your weight gain progress weekly – how much you gained will determine if you need to modify your macros, and if so, which of the macronutrients needs adjustment and by how many grams.

There are various ways to bulk up and gain more muscle, but first you should determine which type of bulk diet you need to gain lean fat – a dreamer bulk, dirty bulk or a lean bulk.

If you choose to get lean fat then you should do a lean bulk. You can do this by increasing your macros for a certain period. You can start with your present macros and increase gradually to your bulk macros. A general guide suggests that you increase your intake by 100 calories per week. Also, increase your fat and protein levels, and then your carbs and other macros.

A lean bulk is the process of increasing your macros to gain more muscle instead of fats. It is the opposite of a dirty bulk. Bulking up does not mean that you literally get bulky. Women are afraid of weight lifting since they mistakenly think that will gain too much muscle and start looking like a man; this kind of thing will not happen naturally. Women do not have testosterone, and this means they will not be able to get muscles that are as large as that of a man's, unless of course they use steroids.

Calculating Total Daily Energy Expenditure (TDEE)

To increase your muscle mass efficiently, you need to calculate your TDEE, and then make sure that you have around 5-15% calorie surplus. You can calculate your TDEE yourself by using various online tools, or you can consult an expert to get a more accurate number.

Using the IIFYM Calculator

Step 1 – Compute your TDEE

Enter your age, weight, height, gender, and workout level. If you are not aware of your body fat percentage, you can also use the Mifflin-St Jeor formula.

Step 2 – Select Your Goals
You can choose from three bulking options – 5% cautious, 10% textbook and 15% aggressive. The percentage shows the increase above your TDEE calories/maintenance.

Step 3 – Nutrition Plan (IIFYM)
In using the IIFYM calculator

- Set protein to one gram per pounds bodyweight (for women)
- Set fat to 0.40 gram per pounds bodyweight (for women)
- The calculator assigns any leftover calories to carbohydrates instantly

Note: to calculate your weight in pounds, divide it by 0.454

Calculate Without IIFYM Calculator

You can also calculate your macros without IIFYM calculator as long as you aware of your maintenance macros. Bear in mind that 1 g of protein and carbohydrates are 4 calories each, and 1 g of fat is worth 9 calories.

1. Calculate (TDEE)
2. Add 5-15% to get bulking calories
3. Calculate protein requirements
4. Calculate fat requirements
5. Assign rest of calories to carbohydrates

Things to Remember

- For fat loss and bulking up (muscle gain), both fats and proteins are very essential. The protein intake may vary between 1.6g – 3g per kilo.

- A big increase in macros may lead to weight gain, which can level out over time. To prevent this, increase macros in small 100-calorie lots.

- Suggested fibre intake for adults is 30 grams. It is not a macronutrient, and does not provide calories. Make sure you are getting 30 grams of fibre each day for better digestion.

- Your macros are calculated per day – it does not matter if you consume them in one meal or three meals or six meals. Nutrient timing is important.

- You are required to recalculate your macros if your weight or exercise level changes or if your body composition modifies.

Chapter 5 - Flexible Diet Myths

When it comes to losing weight "clean eating" continues today, but for some it has to stop. If you are one of the "clean eaters" then you might have made some wrong remark about flexible dieters. Maybe you have even commented on their moral character.

This Chapter discusses some of the common myths about flexible dieters and the way they eat. This will show you the truth about food freedom.

Myth #1 – Flexible Dieters eat a lot of cr*p all day long

This is not possible. Flexible dieting is not about eating unhealthy foods. Flexible dieting is usually comprised of the foods found in the average Western diet, and most of them are not "bad" at all.

Flexible dieting does allow the consumption of junk food, but only at controlled quantities. Portion control, this is very important in flexible dieting. There is a great difference between 1 donut and 12. Make sure you will not abuse this.

Myth #2 – Flexible Dieting is not healthy

This is definitely not true. Many people say that "clean eating" is the only real way to eat healthy. What is healthy about limiting your food intake? Nothing good will ever come out of putting an entire slew of foods out of your regular diet and just restricting yourself to a particular selection of food items.

- Egg whites and oats for breakfast
- White rice, almonds and chicken for lunch.
- Banana and protein shake for post-workout.
- Green beans and Lean beef for dinner
- Cottage cheese and peanut butter before going to bed.

It's a fact that eating a nutrient-dense diet is healthy. However, that is not what "clean eating" is. There is a high connection between binge eating and exclusive eating. This is no coincidence. Studies have shown that as soon as you forbid yourself from a certain kind of food, your desire for it increases –even if you may have never really wanted it before.

As for the first statement – flexible dieting is unhealthy.

What would you think is worse for your health? Eating a bar of chocolate every night (for a total weekly consumption of 7 bars), enjoying every bit of it, and then continue with your life, OR hurriedly eating not just one but 3 whole chocolate bars in single sitting without controlling yourself and then feeling guilty about what you did, which causes you to eat even more? The answer is very clear.

The most important thing to note is that flexible dieters eat the whole food sources not because they have no other choice, but because that is what they decided to eat.

Myth no. 3 – Flexible dieters think that a cheeseburger is the same as a lean cut of steak.

This is not how flexible dieters think.

There are many people with inaccurate understanding about flexible dieting. It's not true flexible dieters think that way. They might be eating burger because they have weighed out their portions. They have probably been eating well the whole day, and have factored the meal into their macros.

Flexible dieters follow the 80/20 rule. They care about their health the same way clean eaters do, but they also understand that to be able to make a lasting lifestyle change, they need to have a sustainable habit.

Chapter 6 - Losing Weight By Tracking Your Macronutrient Intake

There are many diet fads offering several options for those who intend to lose weight. Health conscious individuals can also apply this eating habit into their everyday routines. The IIFYM diet means eating according to your body's daily macronutrient needs.

One of the benefits of IIFYM diet is that it is customizable. It focuses on the fact that every individual has his or her own nutritional needs based not only on the person's goals, but also on his or her genetics, and daily energy expenditure.

Determining the right ratio that will fit your body is not easy, and you may need to go through a bit of trial and error. One of the drawbacks of IIFYM diet is that it does not focus on healthy foods. This type of diet program is for those who have a hard time following strict diets that restrict "bad foods."

The first step in weight loss using your macronutrients is calculating important factors to determine your daily calorie requirements.

Calculate your BMR or Basal Metabolic Rate. You can get your BMR by comparing your weight, age and height against each other. This will help you determine the amount of calories your body spends while at rest.

Next, you will have to use the Harris Benedict Equation to calculate your Total Daily Energy Expenditure (TDEE). To determine an estimate of the amount of calories your body requires based on your daily activity levels.

For those who aim to lose weight, the IIFYM diet suggests subtracting around 15% from your TDEE to determine your daily intake of calorie. If you are aiming to gain muscle it is best that you add anywhere from five to ten percent to your TDEE. This will be your basis in splitting that number between protein, fat and carbohydrates to know your daily macronutrient allotments.

The suggested amount of calories from fat is 25%, from carbs 50% and from protein 25%. You can use several different methods to determine your macronutrient ratios. As stated earlier, you need a series of trial and error before you can find the ratio that works best for you.

Chapter 7 - Basal Metabolic Rate And Flexible Dieting

Basal Metabolic Rate is the same with RMR or Resting Metabolic Rate, but when it comes to flexible dieting it is a little bit different.

It represents the amount of calories your body need to burns at rest. To calculate the exact amount of calories your body need, use the IIFYM BMR calculator. The BMR calculator is different with the TDEE calculator. Hence, if you need to calculate TDEE, do not use the BMR calculator and vice versa.

Many people who are into flexible dieting commit mistake when using the IIFYM BMR calculator to determine the amount of calories they need. This might cause serious calorie deficit that will lead to muscle loss, and delayed fat loss. It may also cause a serious rebound effect, something that most YOYO dieters have encountered. Keep in mind; TDEE and BMR are not the same. Your baseline is BMR. The IIFYM BMR Calculator will only determine the exact amount of calories that your body requires to stay healthy.

If you want to determine how many calories you require to eat to lose weight and burn fat while flexible dieting, don't use the BMR calculator. Use the IIFYM TDEE calculator to calculate your BMR together with other calories you burn during the day. The IIFYM calculator is best for those who are into flexible dieting that is not after gaining muscle and want to concentrate on fat loss.

Chapter 8 - What Is Carb-cycling?

Carb-cyling is a method of losing fats while building or preserving muscle. This involves creating a schedule that alternates high, low and med carb days.

How Carb Cycling Works?

- Rotate through low/no carb, moderate carb, and high carb throughout the week.
- You need high protein intake every day.
- Your fat consumption is inversely related to your carb consumption. For instance, your fat consumption is low, when your carbs are high and vice versa.

The exact procedures vary in terms of specific amount, but all depend on that simple structure. For instance, you may do four low-carb days, then a high-carb day, and then no-carb day and then start all over again.

The theory behind carb cycling is as follows:

Your high-carb day will replenish your muscles glycogen levels and boost your insulin level, which produces anti-catabolic effects. Most procedures suggest that you do your hardest workout on your high-carb day.

Your moderate-carb day provides you plenty of carbs to maintain the amount of glycogen, but does not put you in caloric deficit to result in weight loss. You do your workouts on these days.

Your no and low carb days are those days where you are in a caloric deficit, and where some individuals claim the magic occurs. These are the days where you fool your body into burning fats at a fast rate by keeping low level of insulin. It is most of the time recommended that you employ cardio or rest days for low/ no carb days, however, if you lift more than three days per week, you will need to add one or more of these days.

To answer the question how effective it is:

Carb cycling is very effective in losing fat. Any dietary procedures that puts you in a caloric deficit, regardless if it is a daily or weekly or monthly, will result in weight loss. It does not matter if there is a macronutrient breakdown.

As long as you keep yourself in a caloric deficit, which means you provide your body less energy than it spends- you will lose weight, regardless of whether the energy comes from carbohydrates, fats, or proteins. What makes the carb cycling more appealing is that you don't have to count calories or actually watch what you eat. You just follow a group of simple guidelines about eating plenty of carbohydrates on high days, moderate days and on low or no days.

This style of dieting works perfectly for maintenance, and may work for losing weight to a certain degree, but if you want to get ripped then it is not recommended.

Obtaining below 18-19% body fat for women 8-9% for men requires that you monitor your macronutrient intake closely. You need to determine how much fat, carbohydrate and protein you are eating each day, and you need to control these numbers to provide yourself with enough caloric deficits to continue with your goal of losing fat, but not that much.

Which is better for Weight Loss Carb Cycling or Traditional Dieting?

Those who use carb-cycling diet will normally accelerate their fat loss during low carb days than those who are into the traditional dieting. To explain this claim see example below:

A study done in the University of Pennsylvania, involving 63 obese adults used one of these two methods of dieting:

- A low-carb, high fat, high-protein diet consists of 20g of carbs per day, which slowly decreases until the user attains the target weight.

- A traditional diet usually contains 60% of calories came from carbs, 15% from protein and 25% from fat.

The outcome: the low-carb group shredded more weight in the first three months, but at twelve months, the difference was not significant.

The three-month outcome is not surprising, thinking that lowering carb intake lowers water retention, and also decreases the amount of glycogen stored in muscles and liver, which further reduced the total body water retention.

Another study carried out by Harvard University on diet composition and losing weight. The study involves 811 overweight adults to one of the suggested four diets:

- Twenty percent of calories from fat, fifteen percent from protein, and sixty-five percent from carbs
- Forty percent from fat, fifteen percent from protein, and forty five percent from carbs
- Forty percent from fat, twenty-five percent from protein, and thirty five percent from carbs

The outcome: after six months, participants who lost around 6 kg, start to regain weight after twelve months, and after two years, everyone lost around 4kg. The study concluded that a reduced-calorie diets results in weight loss regardless which macronutrients they focused on.

Therefore, if you want to lose weight, you should choose carb-cycling instead of traditional dieting. This has proven to be very effective several times.

Chapter 9 - Get In Shape Using The IIFYM Calculator

This chapter will explains how you can get in shape using the IIFYM calculator

1. Purchase a digital food scale, to make your diet more effective weigh your uncooked food in grams
2. Open a free online account from the following sources:
   www.myfitnesspal.com
   www.fitday.com
   www.calorieking.com
3. Make use of the IIFYM calculator to calculate the macros that you need based on your body and energy levels.
4. For the first three months weigh everything you eat
5. On your online resource, log everything you eat
6. If you are trying to lose weight, your calorie consumption should be 15-20% less than you're TDEE, every day.
7. If you want to gain weight, eat between five and ten percent more calories than your TDEE, every day.
8. To make sure that you get in shape using IIFYM calculator, follow these steps:

   - Eat at least one gram of protein in every pound of your body weight
   - Eat at least .35 g of fat in every pound of your body weight and around .50 g per pound.
   - Any calories left in your daily total weight will come from carbohydrate
   - Take in twenty to twenty five percent of your body weight in fiber every day.
   - Drink one gallon of water every day aside from other liquid that you consume.

9. As soon as your fat loss stalls, lower your daily intake of carbohydrates by not more than ten grams. Control your macros only when you're fat loss stall for five days or more. If you are still making progress do not reduce carbs or calories. Any modification done should be less, and infrequent.

Choose foods that are rich in vitamins and minerals. As soon as you meet the micronutrient requirement, pick the food you love to eat, while keeping within your personal range of macronutrients.

Conclusion

Thank you again for purchasing this book on "*Flexible Diet: The Flexible Diet Ultimate Guide! - Weight Loss Has Never Been Easier! - Get Lean Fast The Simple Way With This IIFYM Flexible Dieting Guide To Fat Loss Forever*!"

I am extremely excited to pass this information along to you, and I am so happy that you now have read and can hopefully implement these strategies going forward.

I hope this book was able to help you understand IIFYM Flexible Dieting is and how to lose fat forever.

The next step is to get started using this information and to hopefully live a healthier and safe life!

Please don't be someone who just reads this information and doesn't apply it, the strategies in this book will only benefit you if you use them!

If you know of anyone else that could benefit from the information presented here please inform them of this book.

Finally, if you enjoyed this book and feel it has added value to your life in any way, please take the time to share your thoughts and post a review on Amazon. It'd be greatly appreciated!

Thank you and good luck!

Preview Of:

30 Day Kettlebell WOD Exercises!

<u>Kettlebell</u>

Get In Shape Fast With Amazing Russian Kettlebell And Cross Training Workouts!

Introduction

I want to thank you and congratulate you for purchasing the book, *30 Day Kettlebell WOD Exercises!*

This "Kettlebell" book contains proven steps and strategies on how to lose weight and tone your muscles using only the Russian kettlebell.

This book covers all the factors that affect weight loss including workouts, resting and diet. By using the tips suggested in this book, you will be able to lose weight fast without the need for expensive equipment. The kettlebell exercises are really easy and they could also be integrated to the workouts that you are already doing. The nutrition principle suggested by this book follows the Paleo and low carb diet. We hope that you will reach your workout goals by using the tips suggested in this book.

Thanks again for purchasing this book, I hope you enjoy it!

Chapter 1: Workout Principles

There are no shortcuts to losing weight. You have to do your part to be able to achieve your dream body. The amount of work needed will vary depending on your current fitness status and your fitness goals.

Set your Goals

Every important achievement starts with a goal. It will be easier to accomplish your fitness achievement if you also start it with a goal. In stating our goals, we need to make sure that they are specific. It should not be open to any other interpretation. If you aim to lose weight, you should have a number of kilograms or pounds stated in your goal. If it is about having abs, you should measure the diameter of your tummy and you should look for a picture of a fit and toned abs to use as reference.

Your goal should also have a deadline, but make sure that it is realistic. Ensure that you can accomplish your goals according to the deadline that you set. Setting a deadline that is too near will leave you frustrated because you will not be able to reach your goals on time. Setting a deadline that is too far may also lead you to fail. People usually procrastinate when they have too much time to finish a goal.

Lastly, your fitness goals should be reachable based on your resources. You should make sure that you have access to all the things that you need to reach your goals.

People who start working out usually have two common goals in mind; to lose weight and to look good. You should stop and think after this chapter to assess what you want to achieve in getting into the kettlebell WOD program suggested by this book. You should put it into writing and paste it in a place where you will always see it.

Your additional goal:

Aside from your personal goals, it is the duty of every workout mentor to encourage you to keep a healthy lifestyle. After reaching the goals that you set today, you must set more goals to work for.

If you continue to do this, you will be able to make your workouts a part of your lifestyle. By doing this, the fitness accomplishments that you achieve will become permanent. You will have a toned physique and an athletic frame even when you grow older. You will also be able to maintain a healthy weight even as you enter middle age. This is usually the time when people start failing to meet their scheduled workouts and start gaining weight and beer belly.

The Role of Nutrition

Though this book focuses on the workouts, it also teaches the role of nutrition in your weight loss and fitness goals. Just because you workout often doesn't mean that you can eat any type or amount of food that you like. We will discuss the best kind of diet that will best work with your high intensity workouts.

This will be discussed in the later parts of the book.

Thanks for Previewing My Exciting Book Entitled:

"Kettlebell: 30 Day Kettlebell WOD Exercises! Get In Shape Fast With Amazing Russian Kettlebell And Cross Training Workouts!"

To purchase this book, simply go to the Amazon Kindle store and simply search:

"KETTLEBELL"

Then just scroll down until you see my book. You will know it is mine because you will see my name "Chris Smith" underneath the title.

Alternatively, you can visit my author page on Amazon to see this book and other work I have done. Thanks so much, and please don't forget your free bonuses

DON'T LEAVE YET! - CHECK OUT YOUR FREE BONUSES BELOW!

Free Bonus Offer: Get Free Access To The www.LiveFitVIP.com VIP Newsletter!

Once you enter your email address you will immediately get free access to this awesome newsletter!

But wait, right now if you join now for free you will also get free access to the "The 7 Keys To Body Transformation" free EBook!

To claim both your FREE VIP NEWSLETTER MEMBERSHIP and your FREE BONUS Ebook on THE 7 KEYS TO BODY TRANSFORMATION!

Just Go To:

www.liveFitVIP.com